A Christian Woman's Journal to Weight Loss

By Patricia Thomas

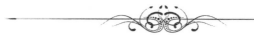

A Christian Woman's Journal to Weight Loss

Published by
The Elevator Group, Faith Imprint
Paoli, Pennsylvania

Copyright © 2009 by Patricia Thomas

ISBN 978-0-9820384-0-6

Jacket and interior design by Stephanie Vance-Patience

Published in the United States by The Elevator Group, Faith Imprint.

This book was printed in the United States.

To order additional copies of this book, contact:
The Elevator Group Faith
PO Box 207
Paoli, PA 19301
www.TheElevatorGroup.com
610-296-4966
info@TheElevatorGroup.com

PERMISSIONS

The following authors, their agents, and publishers have granted permission to include excerpts from the following:

Scripture quotations marked NLT are taken from the Holy Bible, New Living Translation, copyright 1996, 2004. Used by permission of Tyndale House Publishers, Inc., Wheaton, Illinois 60189. All rights reserved.

Scripture taken from the New King James Version. Copyright © 1982 by Thomas Nelson, Inc. Used by permission. All rights reserved.

Scripture taken from the HOLY BIBLE, NEW INTERNATIONAL VERSION®. Copyright © 1973, 1978, 1984 International Bible Society. Used by permission of Zondervan. All rights reserved.

Scriptures marked as CEV are taken from the Contemporary English Version Copyright © 1995 by American Bible Society. Used by permission.

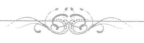

DEDICATION

In loving memory of
My Mother, Lucille Patterson
My Grandmother, Minnie Bridges
The women who allowed me to believe
that anything is possible.

INTRODUCTION

Tired, fatigued, unmotivated, drained, uncomfortable, embarrassed, self-conscious, insecure, ashamed, let-down, disappointed, sad, disgusted, lonely, misunderstood, defeated, miserable, angry, drained, overlooked, side-lined, overweight. These are some of the feelings I had on any given day when I was overweight. Physically, I would often find myself exhausted, not able to do the things I wanted to do. Usually, I would muster up enough energy to meet the obligations and commitments I had made. But, I had no energy left for me. Emotionally, I was so disappointed in myself and sometimes even depressed: how could I let this happen to me? Spiritually, I felt fruitless I was so concerned with my weight that I was not walking in my purpose at all. It is hard to be used by God when you can't see beyond your circumstance.

When I really took the time to analyze my situation, I realized being overweight was about to take me out, emotionally, spiritually, and physically. I was slowly shutting down, but no one knew it. I was able to function everyday as if everything was normal. I am sure I even smiled. I was going through the motions, feeling very empty and robotic. I even remember my doctor saying that my cholesterol was now borderline. Not only did I not want to hear that, I planned to share this new revelation with no one. Normally a healthy person, full of life and filled with the joy of the Lord, this was a new place for me.

There were times when I thought about how things used to be, and I would ask myself: how did I get here? I remembered that I used to have energy to study the word; I used to make the time to spend in prayer. I had lost sight of the importance of spending time with God. I had gotten so caught up in getting through my days, realizing that that was all I was doing—getting through my days. I wasn't living in victory; I wasn't seeking God's face, and I wasn't worshiping outside of church. I was disconnected from the source of my strength, and I was reaping the harvest, which wasn't a very healthy one.

I am not a nutritionist or an expert on health, but I am a woman sharing her true story, giving others a glimpse into the realities of weight loss. My credentials for authoring this book include twelve years of battling with weight and, at 42, finally reaching my goal. After trying diets and weight loss gimmicks, I realized that achieving a positive self image is about so much more than food. I have also realized that women everywhere want to know what is working for other women. So, in January, I decided that I would not only lose the extra pounds, but I would keep a journal of my journey and share it with other women who are also struggling with their weight. Over time, it has developed into a daily devotional that I use to stay focused, encouraged and inspired to make myself a priority.

Like most women who are overweight, I wanted to find a personal solution that worked I wasn't interested in quick-fix drug solutions, and I wanted lasting results. If you are battling with a weight issue, I can only hope that reading this devotional and starting your own weight loss journal, will allow you to experience the fulfillment of achieving a positive self image and your weight loss goal. The benefits of weight loss are priceless. Becoming strong in soul, mind, and body can allow you to reclaim what every woman deserves: her health, her energy, her relationships, her life.

Therefore, if anyone is in Christ, he is a new creation;
the old has gone, the new has come!
—2 Corinthians 5:17

> *I beseech you therefore, brethren, by the mercies of God, that ye present your bodies a living sacrifice, holy, acceptable unto God, which is your reasonable service.*
>
> —Romans 12:1

One of our neighbors was planning a trip, and they asked my family if we would take care of their tadpoles. While our neighbors were away, we made sure we followed all of the care instructions very carefully. We fed them the right amount of food at the right time. We made sure the lighting was adequate and the correct water level was maintained. When our neighbors returned, their tadpoles were healthy frogs that had been well cared for.

In comparison, that week I am sure I ate more than I should have. I probably didn't get enough rest, and I know I didn't exercise at all. Is this how we care for the body that God has entrusted us with?

Yes, all too often, we care for the things around us better than we care for ourselves. How can we present our bodies as a living sacrifice, holy, and acceptable unto God, if we are not at our best? Since I have been overweight, I feel sluggish, frustrated and on edge. Today, I am making a commitment to take care of this body. Being victorious through Christ includes conquering this thing called obesity and living a healthy lifestyle.

It's not just about food; I know this. We all know what we should or shouldn't be eating.

And if we didn't know what to eat, there are hundreds of diet plans out there to tell us. But I don't think I need one. I believe the bigger question is not what we eat, but why, how much, and when?

Today I pledge to care for my body. I know it is going to be a lot of work and even as I write this, I am not looking forward to it. Then I weigh my options. I don't want to continue the cycle of taking care of everything but me. We can get so busy doing things and going places for everyone else that we forget to make time for ourselves. I know this is a journey and I can't expect to see dramatic changes overnight, but I look forward to the small victories that I will experience along the way.

My Pledge to myself:

January 15th 2011 - So many changes have taken place in my life in the past months. My beloved Bonnie died on Dec 7th. I have tried to look out for her for so many years. I feel that I have let my self get lost in all of it. My heart breaks each time I think of her, and the suffering she faced everyday. Her one dream for me was for me to lose weight. She always told me that I had such a pretty face, that she could not believe I had let myself go. When I get stressed out I seem to eat and just retreat into myself. So now I pledge for my self to lose the weight get my self together Not only for my self but for my Bonnie. She is in Gods hand now and I must release her to him and make her proud of me.

WEEK TWO

No temptation has over taken you except such is common to man:
but God is faithful, who will not allow you to be tempted beyond
what you are able, but with the temptation will also make the way of escape,
that you may be able to bear it.
—1 Corinthians 10:13 *(New King James Version)*

How long will we be fooled by the enemy and our flesh? We don't need that extra piece of bread! We can live without that dessert! Now I am not being unrealistic in thinking that I will never enjoy some of the wonderful foods that are available to us, but I know that in my effort to lose weight I have to be able to say "no", and be willing to eat healthier foods. The word tells us that in everything there is a season, and I know that during this season that I am in right now, I have to push away from the table.

I remember being able to eat anything I wanted to and never gaining a pound. Those were the days, but those days are GONE. So, even though I am tempted to continueto eat that way, I know I can not. It is a new day, and my plate has to reflect that.

I am going to look for my way of escape when I am tempted. I give in to temptation more often when I am hungry. I added six glasses of water into my routine today, and I was less tempted. Water can really fill you up.

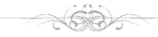

My way of escape will be:

And we know that all things work together for good to them that love God, to them who are called according to His purpose.
—Romans 8:28

Very few things today come with a 'lifetime guarantee', but Christianity does. The word tells us that, all things work together for good to them that love God. This also gives us a clue that every day or every situation isn't going to work out the way we have planned it. There will be those days when we stumble or don't make the best decisions, but it doesn't have to stop there.

Knowing that some days are going to be a real struggle, I am learning to plan for the struggle. As a Christian, we plan for the struggles when we live by the word, so that when trouble comes we can stand. During this weight loss journey we have to do the same thing. We need to be prepared for those tough days when we want to eat everything in sight. Have a plan.

Having meals planned out ahead of time helps me stay on track. I am less likely to make that unhealthy choice if I already know what I am going to eat. I will make it to the gym if I schedule it as a part of my day. As women we plan to get everything else done, we deserve to be on our own schedules.

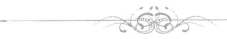

My daily plan:

_____
_____
_____
_____
_____
_____
_____
_____
_____
_____
_____
_____
_____
_____
_____
_____
_____
_____
_____
_____
_____
_____
_____
_____
_____
_____
_____
_____

I can do all things through Christ who strengthens me.
—Philippians 4:13

Remember when Jesus called Peter to walk on water. The scripture says that Peter got out of the boat and walked on the water and he came toward Jesus. It wasn't until he took his mind off Jesus and looked at his circumstances that he began to sink. In spite of his victory, he began to think about the water around him, his limitations. If he had only kept his mind on the limitless ability he has through the power of Jesus Christ.

What are we focusing on? Are we empowering ourselves with our thoughts or are we crippling ourselves? Doubt or a lack of faith can destroy a dream, keep us from achieving our goals and following God's plan for our life. I have tried to lose weight so many times, and eventually doubt crept in. I would begin to think that I would never lose the weight, I would convince myself that I didn't have time to exercise and that I couldn't possibly eat less.

I am not giving in to doubt this time. I know that I can do all things through Christ whostrengthens me, if I just don't give up. When it comes to weight loss, I have decided that faith coupled with works, equals victory. We can get so caught up in what we see today that we don't believe in what tomorrow can bring if we stay committed.

I have decided that working out in the morning is what works best for me. If I don't do it in the morning, my day gets so busy it will not get done. It actually wakes me up and it seems to give me will power throughout the day. I am less tempted to have those chips or waste my workout on a cookie.

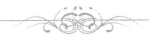

My workout schedule:

_____
_____
_____
_____
_____
_____
_____
_____
_____
_____
_____
_____
_____
_____
_____
_____
_____
_____
_____
_____
_____
_____
_____
_____
_____
_____
_____
_____
_____

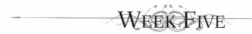

In all thy ways acknowledge Him, and He shall direct thy paths.
—Proverbs 3:6

We have all found ourselves in the middle of a situation alone. We either left God at church on Sunday, we felt that we had the situation under control, or we just weren't in the habit of acknowledging the Lord in all we do. What would happen if we put all things in 'spiritual perspective' before we act?

When did food become so important or begin to play such an big role in our lives?

We use food to nourish our bodies, but we also use it to: celebrate, pamper, soothe us and reward ourselves or others. We can enjoy food, but we have to put it in perspective.

The cravings can be so intense, resisting them seems almost impossible. Isn't it interesting, though, that after we've had the food that we've been craving so much, it doesn't always satisfy the craving? So the question is, what are we really craving?

Instead of having a donut, only to follow that up with some chips or a piece of pie, we need to figure out what we are really craving. This would save us from consuming so many pointless, unnecessary calories.

Today I added sit-ups to my workout. I walk on the treadmill for 45 minutes and I do sit-ups at night before I go to bed. I have noticed that I have more energy when I work out. Now, that's something. We can convince ourselves not to work out because we are too tired when working out actually fuels us with more energy.

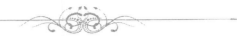

What am I really craving? Can I replace it with something healthy or have it in smaller quantities?

_____

_____

_____

_____

_____

_____

_____

_____

_____

_____

_____

_____

_____

_____

_____

_____

_____

_____

_____

_____

_____

_____

_____

_____

*Jesus said, "Just as I have loved you, you should love each other.
Your love for one another will prove to the world that you are my disciples."*
—John 13:34-35 (NLT)

God knows our heart and how we would respond in certain situations. He knows that some of us could not handle being a size '8', right now. We would be so judgmental of others and act like we have never had a weight problem. "Girl, she just let herself go, she needs to get herself together". We will quickly forget the weight loss challenges we had and have no empathy for what our sister may be going through. God knows we aren't ready until we are comfortable enough with who we are, so we can have a non-judging spirit and be accepting of others.

Years ago before I had a weight problem, I had no idea how hard it was to lose weight. Maybe if I knew how hard it was, I would have been more cautious. It all started for me when I was pregnant with my first child. I was 130 pounds and wearing a size 8 when I first realized I was pregnant. When I went into the delivery room 8 ½ months later, I weighed 210 pounds. Well, the rest is history. The roller-coaster ride started that day. I couldn't blame the weight on my pregnancy anymore.

Not only do we have to learn to love ourselves enough to say 'no', we have to love one another the way God intended. He is holding us accountable, we have to love our sisters and not be so critical of each other.

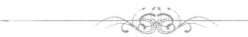

When did my weight loss rollercoaster begin?

_____

_____

_____

_____

_____

_____

_____

_____

_____

_____

_____

_____

_____

_____

_____

_____

_____

_____

_____

_____

_____

_____

_____

_____

_____

_____

_____

_____

I press toward the mark for the prize of the high calling of God in Christ Jesus.
—Philippians 3:14

The scriptures teach us to press our way, and we can't do that if we are looking back or looking down. If we are going to press our way forward, we have to be looking in the right direction.

This is vital when it comes to weight loss. Looking back can cause us to lose our motivation to move forward. We have all done it. We overeat on Friday, so we throw in the towel on Saturday, and the downward spiral begins. This was my biggest challenge. If I messed up, it would take days or weeks for me to get things back under control. I would feel so defeated and go back to my old eating habits, only to find myself starting all over again a few pounds heavier.

We live by grace. If God, who is perfect, can forgive us when we've done wrong, why can't we forgive ourselves and move on? If we overeat on a Friday, let's get up and get right back on track. It doesn't have to turn into an out-of-control eating frenzy.

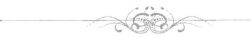

When am I most likely to lose control?

_____

_____

_____

_____

_____

_____

_____

_____

_____

_____

_____

_____

_____

_____

_____

_____

_____

_____

_____

_____

_____

_____

_____

_____

_____

_____

_____

_____

_____

_____

Be anxious for nothing, but in everything by prayer and supplication,
with thanksgiving, let your requests be made known to God; and the
peace of God, which surpasses all understanding, will guard your hearts and
minds through Christ Jesus.
—Philippians 4:6-7 *(New International Version)*

We have become just like the world, a microwave society. We expect everything in seconds. Studies show that if we reduce our food intake and increase our activity, we can expect to lose an average of three pounds a week. So if I want to lose 40 pounds, how can I expect this to happen in three weeks?

Reaching your weight loss goals can take months or years, depending on how much you have to lose. In fact, during the weight loss process, you will probably hit a few plateaus, and this can further reduce your average weekly weight loss. Losing weight is a journey, and you can't expect it to be a mini-excursion.

Our minds must be renewed to look at food differently, view exercise as a vehicle for change, and time as an opportunity for progress. Expecting more than we can possibly deliver in a short period of time will only set us up for failure. Let's be anxious for nothing. What's four months of effort for a lifetime of reward?

I snack heavily between the hours of 7:00pm-9:00pm. I will spend less time in the kitchen during these hours and I will have low calorie snacks available. Losing weight is not rocket science. We all know that we need to eat less and exercise more. The goal is to develop a personal routine that includes healthy lifestyle choices.

I will conquer the temptation to snack by:

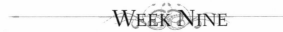
And whatsoever ye do, do it heartily, as to the Lord, and not unto men;
—Colossians 3:23

I hate feeling uncomfortable in my clothes. It's like a vicious cycle. I don't want to buy bigger sizes, but a lot of the clothes that I have don't fit quite right. So there are many days when I wear something that isn't very comfortable. In fact, I remember one Sunday in church not wanting to stand because I felt my skirt was a little tight.

I believe that not feeling good about how we look has an impact in every aspect of our life. We can't be all that God wants us to be if we are not comfortable in our own skin. Our weight could be holding us back from experiencing our full potential. God deserves our best and so do we. It's time for a change.

It is a good feeling to know that I can do something about my weight and each day there is a little less of me. Finding ways to encourage ourselves during this journey will help keep us motivated. Today I rewarded myself with a manicure. When I feel good about myself, I find that I am less likely to grab that fat-filled, high calorie snack.

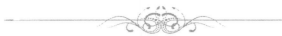

I will encourage and reward myself with:

_____

_____

_____

_____

_____

_____

_____

_____

_____

_____

_____

_____

_____

_____

_____

_____

_____

_____

_____

_____

_____

_____

_____

_____

_____

_____

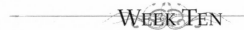

Let your moderation be known unto all men. The Lord is at hand.
—Philippians 4: 5

Pray for a balanced life. We have become over-worked, over-booked, over-loaded and over-eaters. More, more, more, more seems to be the trend. We work more, we juggle more, we spend more, we eat more. Should we really have anything we want, when we want it, without constraint?

Restaurants are trying to satisfy this need we have for more by offering, super sizes and " all- you- can- eat" options. Neither of these promote a healthy lifestyle. Now everyone may want to enjoy a Biggie Fry every now and then, but overindulging on a regular basis is not what our bodies are equipped to handle.

Years ago we weren't so obese as a nation. Family values is what drove the family, not schedules and activities. We had time to prepare more balanced meals. A balanced lifestyle will help us balance our food intake. We are even passing this unbalanced lifestyle to the next generation. Our children are becoming overbooked, and the USDA reports that 27 percent of our children are overweight.

As women, I think it is in our nature to say yes. I knew I was over committed when I didn't have time to cook or do laundry. Something had to give. I reevaluated my schedule. I don't think anyone benefits if we are running all over town day after day giving what's left of ourselves, versus trimming our schedule and giving our best to a few things.

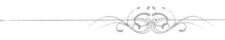

I will balance my life by:

_____

_____

_____

_____

_____

_____

_____

_____

_____

_____

_____

_____

_____

_____

_____

_____

_____

_____

_____

_____

_____

_____

_____

_____

_____

_____

_____

_____

This book of the law shall not depart out of thy mouth; but thou shalt meditate therein day and night, that thou mayest observe to do according to all that is written therein: for then thou shalt make thy way prosperous, and thou shalt have good success.
—Joshua 1:8

God has a way of making things very clear. He can open our eyes, allowing us to see and put things in perspective. When I start my day with Him, I am more in control of my day, my tasks don't seem so monstrous and food seems so insignificant in comparison with my desire to please Him. Notice I said, when I start my day with Him.

This journey is a battle. We are fighting against the will of the flesh daily. I know in my heart, soul and mind that starting my day in devotion centers my day, yet time constraints and fatigue can be allowed to minimize the need for this all important quiet time.

I am determined that I can not, and I will not, allow the pressures of this world to steal my communion with the Lord. I had to decide that no matter what is going on in my life, the One who gave me life will be Lord of my life. My time with Himis no longer optional.

Spending time studying the word and time in prayer is not for God's benefit. He reminds us to do these things because He wants us to live in victory. When we go through our day without Him, it's like trying to maneuver through a room in the dark. We would decrease our chances of falling if we had just turned on the light.

My precious time with the Lord will be:

_____
_____
_____
_____
_____
_____
_____
_____
_____
_____
_____
_____
_____
_____
_____
_____
_____
_____
_____
_____
_____
_____
_____
_____
_____
_____
_____

WEEK TWELVE

I hope that you are as strong in body as I know you are in spirit.
—3 John: 2 (CEV)

Don't skip a meal. Give your body what it needs. We know that we are healthiest when we eat three well balanced meals a day. Trying to starve ourselves is unhealthy and we've all tried it, but it doesn't work. If we start skipping meals we usually give in to temptation eventually because we are so hungry.

Although we are trying to lose weight, we shouldn't walk around hungry. We can only operate that way in the short run. If you're like me and you have a lot of weight to lose, it's going to take a while, and no one will stick to a reduced calorie diet if they're hungry.

Also, in order for our bodies to function properly, we have to feed it. You know our mood even changes when we get hungry. Some of us do not need to be around other people when our stomachs are growling. We can get a little snippy. A lack of food impacts how we operate. It's just like a machine: no juice, no power.

I eat three meals a day. I typically eat cereal and fruit for breakfast, a low calorie frozen food entree for lunch, and a sensible dinner. If I need a snack, I have been having popcorn, veggies or 100 calorie snack packs. I may switch it up a little bit when I get bored, but the key for me has been planning. Having the right snacks available and leaving a lot of things in the store. If it's in the kitchen, I can be tempted to eat it.

But, if it's at the store, chances are very slim that I will run to the store to satisfy a craving.

My daily food plan will consist of:

_____

_____

_____

_____

_____

_____

_____

_____

_____

_____

_____

_____

_____

_____

_____

_____

_____

_____

_____

_____

_____

_____

_____

_____

_____

_____

The thief cometh not, but for to steal, and to kill, and to destroy: I am come that they might have life, and that they might have it more abundantly.
—John 10:10

Being mindful of what we eat, getting enough exercise and making sure our body is healthy is very important, but we don't have to obsess about it. God's plan includes us enjoying life, not being anxious about it. As we work to become a healthier person inside and out, we shouldn't stop living.

In the past when I have tried to lose weight, I think the feeling of deprivation also attributed to me not reaching my goal. I was so obsessed with the fact that I was dieting, that I walked around with the sense that I was missing out. And when we feel that something is being withheld from us, what to we do? Well, we are going to find a way to get it.

When we are eating healthier, what are we really being deprived of? Sugar, saturated fat and carbohydrates? When we look at it in those terms, it doesn't seem so appealing. In fact, I am consuming all of these, but just not in excessive amounts. When we are trying to lose weight, obsessing about it can be defeating.

Today, I look at my lifestyle change with a new perspective. I am eating healthy, not dieting. I am choosing to watch my sugar, fat and carbohydrate intake. I am not being forced. I enjoy having more energy, and I look forward to the reward that will come from hard work and determination. And I am not expecting this reward next week!

My new perspective on food is:

_____

_____

_____

_____

_____

_____

_____

_____

_____

_____

_____

_____

_____

_____

_____

_____

_____

_____

_____

_____

_____

_____

_____

_____

_____

WEEK FOURTEEN

Be on guard and stay awake. Your enemy, the devil, is like a roaring lion, sneaking around to find someone to attack. But you must resist the devil and stay strong in your faith. You know that all over the world the Lord's followers are suffering just as you are.
—1 Peter 5:8-9 (CEV)

Wake up! What am I doing battling with a donut? When I went grocery shopping, I used to get a donut to eat as I shopped. Not just a regular donut either. It was an apple fritter. It's at least 500 calories. I can't keep doing this. The battle is not with the fritter. It's with my flesh. Discipline is a key component of Christianity and the cornerstone of a successful weight loss plan.

Habits are hard to break, so we just have to develop new ones. The foods we enjoy are never going to go away. They will always be available. So let's face it. If we don't learn to kick the habit of over eating or over indulging, the weight loss battle will never end. If we have always had a snack before bed, kick that habit and have a small desert after dinner instead. It's better to eat at 6:00 p.m. as opposed to 9:30 p.m. If we normally eat at our desk all day, try drinking at our desk all day. You know what I mean, get some bottles of water or diet soda.

I try not to go to the grocery store hungry, and I shop better with a grocery list. Now, I am less likely to make choices that will come back to haunt me later. Also, when I am buying snacks for my girls and my husband, I choose snacks from their list that are not appealing to me.

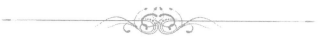

I can change my grocery store experience by:

_____

_____

_____

_____

_____

_____

_____

_____

_____

_____

_____

_____

_____

_____

_____

_____

_____

_____

_____

_____

_____

_____

_____

_____

_____

But they that wait upon the Lord shall renew their strength; they shall mount up with wings as eagles; they shall run and not be weary; and they shall walk, and not faint.
—Romans 41:31

What do we do while we wait? We have all found ourselves in a situation where we have had to wait on God. I believe our response from God can be determined by what we do while we are waiting. As we wait for an answer to prayer, are we acting on faith? Are our actions in line with the word? If we are waiting on God to bless us with that new job, are we working as unto the Lord on the job we have? He is a gracious God, and he wants to bless us. I believe our blessings come when our lives mirror the word, which is a blueprint of the life God has planned for us.

Waiting. What we do while we are waiting to reach our weight loss goal also determines if or when we reach our goal. The wait may be long and there is so much that we have to do to get there, so what do we do while we wait? I had to find ways to enjoy my journey. Sometimes I would try on clothes that used to fit, but now they are a little lose. I also try on clothes that I want to wear when I reach my goal. I am sure we all have those closets of all sizes, and we can use this to our advantage. I am encouraged when I spend a little time noticing my progress and anticipating future successes.

Signs of weight loss motivate me. I also enjoy pampering myself. Whether it be a facial, a movie, a pedicure or a new hair cut, it's a healthy pick-me-up.

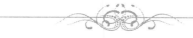

While I'm waiting I will:

_____

_____

_____

_____

_____

_____

_____

_____

_____

_____

_____

_____

_____

_____

_____

_____

_____

_____

_____

_____

_____

_____

_____

_____

_____

_____

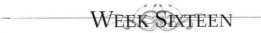

Endurance develops strength of character in us.
—Romans 5:4 (NLT)

Most of us who have dieted before can agree there is a honeymoon period. Oh, the first week we watch what we eat, and we are filled with excitement and expectancy.

Now, by week 10, 7, or even week 3, the zeal is gone. We don't want to see another veggie, the thought of water makes us gag, and visions of an ice cream sundae or a slice of cheesecake are hard to resist. We want to be at our goal, but now the effort needed to get there seems like just too much.

If only we could bottle the zeal from the first week and carry it with us throughout our weight loss journey, I believe we would get to our goal much sooner. The definition for the word *endure* is "to put up with something for a long time." We are really experts at this skill. Some of us find it hard to get up when that alarm rings, but we do it. Who likes folding clothes or mopping, but we do it. We put up with so much, for reasons less important than losing weight. We now need to apply that enduring spirit to our weight loss efforts.

A friend of mine shared a phrase with me that I have used to motivate me when I have considered giving up. She said, "Skinny tastes better than food". It doesn't work all the time, but it can motivate you to pass on that second helping of potatoes or that piece of bread with butter.

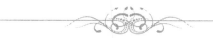

When I consider giving up I will:

_____

_____

_____

_____

_____

_____

_____

_____

_____

_____

_____

_____

_____

_____

_____

_____

_____

_____

_____

_____

_____

_____

_____

_____

_____

_____

_____

_____

WEEK SEVENTEEN

Now faith is the substance of things hoped for, the evidence of things not seen.
—Hebrews 11:1

The Word tells us to act on what we believe, not necessarily what we see, think, or feel. This is so true with weight loss. You really have to rely on faith during this journey.

There are times when it doesn't seem as if you are making any progress. You know what happens then; the motivation to continue dissipates. No one wants to struggle for nothing. And that is what the enemy would like you to believe is happening right now. Nothing. Yes, the enemy doesn't want you to reach your goal. He has a vested interest in you staying defeated, frustrated and discouraged.

When it doesn't seem like anything is happening, this is the time to plant your feet and stand. I believe God is at work when we get to the "seems like" in our situation. If you haven't, you surely know of someone who has experienced God's hand during this time. During a routine checkup in 2005, my blood work results showed something irregular. My doctor called me and scheduled an appointment with a hematologist. A little shaken, my husband and I went to see this doctor. He explained to us the potential of a blood disorder and said that he was going to run additional tests. While it seemed like there was an issue, God was working it out. The results from the second test confirmed that I was in good health.

During my weight loss this time, I am not going to respond based on what seems to be happening. If I am working out, eating right and taking care of myself, that in itself is progress (even if the scale doesn't show it). And if it doesn't look like victory today,

I know if I continue in faith, the scale will eventually tip in my favor.

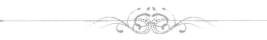

When it doesn't seem like anything is happening I will:

What? Know you not that your body is the temple of the Holy Spirit
which is in you, which ye have of God, and you are not your own?
For you are bought with a price: thereforeglorify God in your body, and in
your spirit, which are God's.
—1 Corinthians 6:19-20

We are fearfully and wonderfully made. When God created us, He created a temple that proclaims His sovereignty. The human body is a masterpiece, our hearts circulate blood through the body about 1000 times a day. We have six muscles just in our face. The small intestine is 22 feet long, tucked neatly in place. Our brain is made up of 10 billion nerve cells and weighs less than three pounds. The list of amazing facts about our bodies is endless. Taking care of what we have been blessed with shouldn't not be an after thought, but a lifetime commitment.

Variety is good when you are working out and eating. Eating the same old thing or doing the same old thing can get boring, and we will find ourselves doing and eating other things. Have you ever found yourself standing with the refrigerator or cupboard open, just looking for something else to eat? This is dangerous. You can find yourself picking several things that you should have right now.

I found a way to spice up my salads because they were getting a little boring. I added smoked salmon on top with a few nuts. It was really delicious. I am not fond of rice cakes, but when you top them with some flavor, they aren't too bad. I add tuna made with low fat mayonnaise, or sometimes I have them with Nutella on top when I want something sweet.

I have also been mixing up my workout routine. I will either walk on the treadmill, use the stepper, or the elliptical. I enjoyed the change. It makes the time go faster, and I feel better about going to the gym. Change works for me.

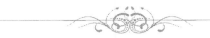

I will add variety to my weight loss by:

To be comforted by God, what a thought. I say a "thought", because most of us don't take the time to be comforted by God. We look for comfort in many other places, only to continue our search. Spending time with God offers a peace that is indescribable. Instead of looking for comfort in all the wrong places, we can have a little talk with the Lord and have the faith to rely on Him. Doing this can bring us to a comforting place of rest.

I have to acknowledge that I don't just eat to satisfy a craving or out of enjoyment. I have learned that I eat for many other reasons. As I have been journaling, I have been more cognizant of when I eat and why. I eat when I am tired and I can't lay down. I eat when I have had a rough day and I am upset. I even eat if I have work to do and I am avoiding getting started. During these times, I can find myself walking around the kitchen, looking for something to eat.

We have to listen to our bodies and respond accordingly to what's really going on. Grabbing food as a cure-all for our issues or ailments is a very self destructive habit.

Not only does it not solve the problem (what ever it is), it creates a new one. Maybe we need to talk with someone about our day, unwind with a cup of tea or take a nap instead.

My goal is to limit the amount of time I spend in the kitchen. If I am not cooking or cleaning up in there, I need to get out. I am also learning to relax. I sit in the den more, and I am reading more, and I spend more one on one time with my family.

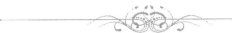

I eat when I:

_____

_____

_____

_____

_____

_____

_____

_____

_____

_____

_____

_____

_____

_____

_____

_____

_____

_____

_____

_____

_____

_____

_____

_____

_____

_____

_____

_____

WEEK TWENTY

*That everyone of you should know how to possess his vessel in
sanctification and honor.*
—1 Thessalonians 4:4

God wants to help us live in a way that is honorable and pleasing to Him. Think about it—what a blessing to have the One who separated night and day, the One who gathered the waters allowing land to appear, the One who breathed life into man, being mindful of our daily needs and circumstances. He will create in us a clean heart and renew a right spirit within us, if we would only ask.

My cholesterol is borderline, so my doctor checks it periodically to make sure it's going in the right direction. This is another reason for me to renew my mind and think of food in a different way. I am not on medication, and I want it to stay that way as long as possible. A healthy lifestyle is a new way of life for me.

Yesterday, I was scheduled for my routine blood work, and you know you can't eat after a certain time in the evening the day before the tests. I thought about how I never have a problem not eating in the evenings when these tests are, scheduled. So I asked myself, "Who said that an evening snack was mandatory"? It's so funny; we are really creatures of habit. If this is the way we've always done it, well this is the way we are going to continue to do it.

For more years than I choose to count, I have given my girls an evening snack, and then I have an evening snack as well. Like clockwork, it's a part of our day. Now, being realistic, I am not saying that I will never have an evening snack, especially on movie night. But, if I have a snack two nights a week as opposed to seven nights, that's an improvement.

The habits that I can rethink are:

_____

_____

_____

_____

_____

_____

_____

_____

_____

_____

_____

_____

_____

_____

_____

_____

_____

_____

_____

_____

_____

_____

_____

_____

Forasmuch then as Christ hath suffered for us in the flesh, arm yourself likewise with the same mind: for he that hath suffered in the flesh hath ceased from sin; That he no longer should live the rest of his time in the flesh to the lusts of men, but to the will of God.
—1 Peter 4:1,2

Having the mind of Christ, this is the goal of Christians. Can you imagine living each day in the perfect will of God? Living to glorify Him and not ourselves or other? Can we glorify Him in our Church, our home and on our jobs? If we are willing to deny the flesh, have a true desire to please Him, and couple that with faith in His word, we can.

There are a lot of things that are good for us that don't taste good, that aren't comfortable, and that may be very unappealing. Like mammograms, spinach, vitamins, exercising, root canals, and the list can go on and on. But just because something doesn't taste good or feel good, doesn't mean we can or should avoid it.

Final exams can be painful, but they are essential to a person's educational success. They may not be the highlight of our year but, wellness checkups are a key component of our overall physical health. Choosing what is easy or comfortable isn't always what's best for us.

I knew losing weight wouldn't be a walk in the park for me. I grew up eating anything I wanted with no concern for weight or health, and now after 30 years I am supposed to watch what I eat! It is hard work for me. I have to accept that, roll up my sleeves and get to work. It will require me eating things that may not be on my list of favorite foods, getting out of my comfort zone and going to the gym.

It may be uncomfortable, but I will:

_____

_____

_____

_____

_____

_____

_____

_____

_____

_____

_____

_____

_____

_____

_____

_____

_____

_____

_____

_____

_____

_____

_____

_____

Let us consider one another in order to stir up love and good works, not forsaking the assembling of ourselves together, as is the manner of some, but exhorting one another, and much the more as you see the Day approaching.
—Hebrews 10:24-25 *(New King James Version)*

In a world where we are not expected to be our brother's/sister's keeper, as Christians we are called to be just that. It takes a power beyond our own to bless those who curse you and do good to those who persecute you. As Christians, we have the power that will enable us to love.

Although we would like to believe it isn't true, everyone doesn't have our best interest at heart. There are those who we allow to get under our skin and who are more effective at tearing us down as opposed to lifting us up. Since my mood can have a direct impact on my will-power, I have to guard it. I just can't let certain people get close enough to do damage.

Yes, we assemble to lift up and to edify, but with some individuals we have to make the assembly brief. You know what I mean. For our own well being, we have to make this choice. We don't lash back or become bitter. We just love them while we are together and minimize contact.

I had to learn to avoid situations that upset me. There's nothing wrong with protecting yourself. I also had to learn not to let external forces determine my mood. The choir at our church sings a song that says, "the joy of the Lord is my strength". Remembering this allows me to get off the emotional roller-coaster and at least reduce the need for comfort food.

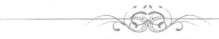

I will protect myself by:

_____

_____

_____

_____

_____

_____

_____

_____

_____

_____

_____

_____

_____

_____

_____

_____

_____

_____

_____

_____

_____

_____

_____

_____

_____

_____

_____

_____

_____

Week Twenty-Three

Your ears shall hear a word behind you, saying, "This is the way, walk in it,"
whenever you turn to the right hand or whenever you turn to the left.
—Isaiah 30:21 *(New King James Version)*

There is something about being full. If we are filled with the Spirit of the living God, there are some things we just won't do. Being filled allows us as Christian's to differentiate right from wrong and honor God in our actions. Discernment is a byproduct of being filled.

The other day at lunch, I was prepared to eat what I had packed and two cookies that were given to me by a child at the school. The cookies looked so good, I actually made a conscious decision to have them with my lunch that day. But myplans changed. My husband met me for lunch and brought me a sub sandwich which was in line with my diet and it was more filling than what I had packed. After eating the sandwich, I didn't even want the cookies anymore. I gave them to my husband and enjoyed the sense of accomplishment I felt. I was full and satisfied, so I didn't need the cookies.

I need will-power like that everyday. I try to avoid being hungry by eating plenty of the things that are good for me, drinking plenty of water, and having healthy snacks readily available.

I will avoid being hungry by:

_____

_____

_____

_____

_____

_____

_____

_____

_____

_____

_____

_____

_____

_____

_____

_____

_____

_____

_____

_____

_____

_____

_____

_____

_____

_____

_____

_____

_____

WEEK TWENTY-FOUR

Whether therefore you eat, or drink, or whatsoever you do, do all to the glory of God.
—1 Corinthians 10:31

Doing all to the Glory of God. In an ordinary day how often do we give thought to glorifying God in all that we do. I think if we were honest, we would admit that a lot of what we do is based on how we feel or what we want. As Christians we are called to test our thoughts and actions. Why do we do what we do?

I remember as a little girl, being told I had to eat everything that was on my plate. I never finished all of my food, and I was always the last one to finish eating. In fact, I would have to sit at the dinner table well past dinner. This was my Mom's attempt to get me to eat. I even started hiding my food so I could get up.

It's kind of ironic, now as an adult, I am usually the first one to finish eating. And as an adult, I eat everything on my plate and more. So I was thinking, why don't I try a smaller plate? This will help regulate my portion size. Now the need to eat everything on my plate is not so bad.

It feels good to be in control of my portions as opposed to being controlled by the food I eat. I don't eat from a saucer everyday, but I use this option when I feel I need it.

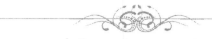

I will control my portions by:

_____

_____

_____

_____

_____

_____

_____

_____

_____

_____

_____

_____

_____

_____

_____

_____

_____

_____

_____

_____

_____

_____

_____

_____

_____

_____

_____

_____

I can do all things through Christ which strengtheneth me.
—Philippians 4:13

If we have the power in us to slay a giant (like David), surely we can defeat obesity.

The story clearly explains the David was out of his league when he went up against Goliath, but David knew the power of the Lord was with him. David went before the giant without the armor that was provided for him. And he said these words to Goliath, "You comest to me with a sword, and with a spear, and with a shield: but I come to thee in the name of the Lord of hosts".

We read about this power. We hear about it every Sunday. But do we receive it? That's the question. Think about it. We are allowing two inches of our body to be in control of the decisions we make. Should we give our mouths that much authority? If we could just find a way to control our lips, we could control our weight.

If food is my Goliath, I can consider what David did to slay his giant. He first acknowledged his opponent. Then he prepared for battle. David had a plan. David didn't get to close to his opponent, he launched his attach from a distance. Lastly David was not overwhelmed by the size of his opponent. In spite of his opponent's stature, he used what he had in the most effective way possible.

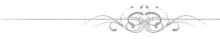

My Goliath is? I will defeat my Goliath by:

_____

_____

_____

_____

_____

_____

_____

_____

_____

_____

_____

_____

_____

_____

_____

_____

_____

_____

_____

_____

_____

_____

_____

_____

_____

_____

_____

_____

_____

_____

WEEK TWENTY-SIX

*Call to Me, and I will answer you, and show you great and mighty things,
which you do not know.*
—Jeremiah 33:3 *(New King James Version)*

What do we pray for? Is it important to pray for self control and physical well-being? Absolutely. A lack of discipline and illness can both hinder us from being all that God wants us to be. Remember, God wants us to have life, and have it more abundantly, and being unnecessarily obese is not living the abundant life.

I don't know who I was fooling all these years. I would never admit it, but I had gotten big, and it was holding me back. I buried myself in other things so I wouldn't have to deal with it. I was busy with the kids, making sure the house was in order, and I was a mess. Where is the victory in that?

Now my day is very different. I spend time in the word when I get up. Then I work out (at least three times a week), and then I start my day. When I decided to make myself a priority, nothing suffered. It's funny; when we are so busy doing who knows what, the thought of adding something else to our day is unthinkable. But, when we get ourselves together, things have a way of falling into place.

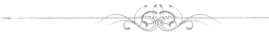

I am praying for:

Through the Lord's mercies we are not consumed, because His compassions fail not. They are new every morning; great is Your faithfulness.
—Lamentations 3:22-23 *(New King James Version)*

If our Father who is perfect can forgive us, can we justify not showing mercy towards others or ourselves? In fact, if we can not forgive, are we thinking more highly of ourselves than we should? We can't forget, all have sinned and fallen short of the glory of God.

If you fall down, get right back up. Everyone has heard this and many of us have told someone this. Well, when you are trying to lose weight every now and then you have to tell yourself. No matter how much support we do or do not have, we must learn to support ourselves. You should always be there for you.

We had family visiting for the week, and although I planned to watch my food intake, it didn't quite work. My weaknesses were the cake and the macaroni and cheese. When you are losing weight, you can't avoid gatherings and celebrations. It's unrealistic to think every day will be a sugar-free day.

So, although I ate some things that I wouldn't normally have eaten, I watched my portions, drank my water and exercised. I didn't feel defeated—just human. When the week was over, things got back to normal with very little damage.

I will support myself by:

You are a chosen generation, a royal priesthood, a holy nation, His own special people, that you may proclaim the praises of Him who called you out of darkness into His marvelous light.
—1 Peter 2:9 *(New King James Version)*

Who do you say you are? Who does the enemy say you are? Who does God say you are? God says you are a conqueror. He says you are like a tree planted by the riverside. He said you have the power to move mountains. If this is truly who we are, are we living the victorious life that God has planned for us?

When we have thoughts that tell us, "I have too much weight to lose", "I can't stick with it", or "I am always going to be overweight"; we have to ask ourselves, " Who am I going to listen to?" Will I believe the words of my Creator or the lies of the enemy? Well I don't know about you but, I choose to believe that I am royal, chosen and special.

When we realize who we are in the Lord, we can make some unusual and peculiar choices. Instead of having that high calorie, fat filled lunch, I can make a different choice. If I have always taken a nap after dinner, I can choose to take a walk instead.

I don't have to do what I've always done. In fact, it takes a new action to achieve a new result.

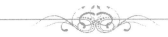

My new action will be:

Do not become sluggish, but imitate those who through faith and patience inherit the promises.
—Hebrews 6:12 *(New King James Version)*

Getting something for nothing, expecting to receive without giving, or having a "what's in it for me" attitude. We all know these thoughts are not biblical. The Word actually says that if you don't work, you shouldn't eat. To enjoy the promises of God, we must roll up our sleeves and be willing to do our part.

Why is it so hard to say, "no"? When we are around foods we know we shouldn't have, it is so easy to give in. We take that first bite, then another and another.

It makes us feel good for a moment, it soothes us, and gives us pleasure. But, that feeling is so temporary. The long term effect of overeating is what is lasting.

In our head, we know we have to begin making choices that are going to benefit us for the long run, not settle for a temporary fix.

In a perfect world, we would only have foods around us that are healthy and good for us, but we are bombarded with high calorie food options that are not sound food choices. We have to decide that we are more important than a slice of bread.

We need to love ourselves more than chocolate syrup.

Honestly, I get more long-term pleasure from a massage than from a piece of cake, from a pedicure versus a bag of chips, or a manicure over a couple of cookies. I have found that reading a magazine with a cup of tea is a great end to my day as opposed to that brownie with ice cream.

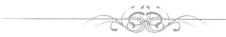

I will find pleasure in:

_____

_____

_____

_____

_____

_____

_____

_____

_____

_____

_____

_____

_____

_____

_____

_____

_____

_____

_____

_____

_____

_____

_____

_____

_____

_____

_____

_____

_____

_____

God saw everything that He had made, and indeed it was very good.
—Genesis 1:31

To be used by God (and that is our goal), we have to be able to look beyond self in order to serve. It is vital that we become comfortable with who we are, so we can focus on other things. When we are worried about our weight and are self-conscious about how we look, it holds us back.

When we look at the big picture, it's not just about losing weight. It's about becoming who we are in Christ. Hebrews 12:1 says, "let us lay aside every weight, and the sin which doth so easily beset us, and let us run with patience the race that is set before us". If there is anything that is restraining us, we must let it go.

I count it a blessing to be able to look at food in a whole new way. It's almost like I was addicted to eating and the consequences of my habit were destroying who I was. The word provides clarity and allows me to see through the sugar.

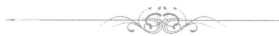

I will lay aside my weight and focus on:

WEEK THIRTY-ONE

She girds herself with strength, and strengthens her arms.
—Proverbs 31:17 (*New King James Version*)

There are many things that can rob us of our strength to resist temptation. Stress, fatigue and hunger are a few of them. Taking care of our bodies involves a lot more than food. Our overall well-being includes our spiritual, emotional, financial and physical health.

We live in a fast-paced world. Trying to do more with less, meeting overly-aggressive deadlines, and keeping up with the Joneses has an effect on our overall wellness. Who decided that we need to stretch our day, our money, or ourselves? Why can't we be who we are, only spend what we can afford, and get done what the day allows? No one should strive to be mediocre, but who benefits from trying to maintain a pace that is self destructive?

I've done it. My motto used to be, "I give 210%." For what! So I can say, I did it?

That is definitely not the Spirit. If we are living an unbalanced life, just to say look what I did, our priorities are all messed up. I am comfortable with giving 100% of me, so that I can do just that, give. Give to the Lord, to my family, my church, and my community. With giving 100%, I also have enough energy left to take care of me.

I will readjust my schedule by:

_____

_____

_____

_____

_____

_____

_____

_____

_____

_____

_____

_____

_____

_____

_____

_____

_____

_____

_____

_____

_____

_____

_____

_____

_____

_____

*And Mary said, My soul magnifies the Lord, and my spirit has
rejoiced in God my Savior.*
—Luke 1:46-47 *(New King James Version)*

God is such a good God. His mercies are new each day. He loves us unconditionally in spite of ourselves, and He has given us His word by which to live an abundant life.

The list of God's goodness can go on and on, culminating with the gift of salvation. Who could not worship such a God as this?

I am thankful today, I am really beginning to notice my weight loss and I thank God for a mind and a desire to become healthier. I look at my former way of thinking as crippling. Thinking that I didn't have a choice and that this was just the way it was going to be was not of God, and I am blessed to know differently.

Usually, when I start to see results I get comfortable and begin to rebound. But not this time. I am going to press my way through and not settle for less than what I deserve. My energy is up, my clothes are starting to fit better, and I am happier. I am not going to give this up. For what, a hot fudge sundae? I don't think so.

God's goodness is evident in my life by:

_____
_____
_____
_____
_____
_____
_____
_____
_____
_____
_____
_____
_____
_____
_____
_____
_____
_____
_____
_____
_____
_____
_____
_____
_____
_____
_____
_____
_____
_____

WEEK THIRTY-THREE

She seeks wool and flax, and willingly works with her hands.
—Proverbs 31:13 *(New King James Version)*

Routine and discipline are a vital part of this Christian walk. When the word speaks of us "taking up our cross and following Him", we know that we are no longer free to live any old way. Living by the word may be challenging, but if we keep reading, we will find out that we win!

Routine and discipline are also two things that I have had to learn to include in my weight loss plan. I am a very routine person, and I can be very disciplined, but in the past I had not really applied it to my weight loss effort. Sticking to something for a couple of weeks really doesn't require much control.

As mothers, we have to be good at juggling family, work schedules, and other responsibilities. This just comes with the territory. It's like trial by fire. There is no time to practice. You are immediately expected to be a master planner, be disciplined, and have a sound routine in place to get through the day.

I applied these skills I've learned as a wife and mother to my personal weight loss goal. It works. I am now on that daily priority list, and I get checked off at the end of the day just like everything else. I am at soccer practice whether I feel like it or not, and now I am at the gym whether I feel like it or not. Now that statement is within reason. There are extreme circumstances when any item on the list can get vetoed if needed. We are all human and need balance.

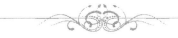

My priority list includes:

_____

_____

_____

_____

_____

_____

_____

_____

_____

_____

_____

_____

_____

_____

_____

_____

_____

_____

_____

_____

_____

_____

_____

_____

_____

_____

_____

_____

_____

_____

_____

_____

WEEK THIRTY-FOUR

Therefore let us pursue the things which make for peace and the things by which one may edify another.
—Romans 14:9 *(New King James Version)*

No matter how dedicated we are to our goal of losing weight, we've had those days when we feel down or defeated. We are tired of the wait and tired of the weight.

Maybe it was a day or a weekend when we ate more that we should have, and will-power seems well beyond our reach. Maybe we are just running low on motivation.

There are numerous scriptures in the word that remind us to encourage or edify each other. We know that nothing in the word is there by coincidence, but purposeful instruction meant for our good. So this tells me that God knows that we have those days when we will need a little encouragement from a friend.

Although I am on this weight loss journey alone, I think it would have been nice to have had a weight loss partner. I think it would have been a little easier. You would have someone to talk with who knows what you're experiencing and who could pump you up when you're running a little low on air.

_____ *could be my weight loss partner because:*

_____

_____

_____

_____

_____

_____

_____

_____

_____

_____

_____

_____

_____

_____

_____

_____

_____

_____

_____

_____

_____

_____

_____

_____

_____

_____

Where there is no vision, the people perish:
but he that keepeth the law, happy is he.
—Proverbs 29: 18

"What You Don't Know Won't Hurt You." Where did that phrase come from? If you don't know, you better ask somebody. The more we know, the more we can apply truth to our lives. Our Bibles should not serve as decoration, but our tool for direction in our daily life. Knowledge is definitely power. It strengthens who we are. It culminates growth.

Did you know that lifting weights in addition to aerobic activity can greatly enhance your workout? Lifting weight builds muscle, and the more muscle we have, the more fat we burn. I think I had heard this before, but I didn't know enough about it to actively add weight lifting into my workout routine.

I used to be uncomfortable using the weights at the gym. It seemed like those were reserved for body building or something. Most of the people using the weights looked like serious body builders. Well, now I use weights and I am excited to see the results.

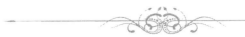

To enhance my weight loss efforts I could learn about:

*And Jesus went about all the cities and villages, teaching in
their synagogues, and preaching the gospel of the
kingdom, and healing every sickness and every
disease among the people.*
—Matthew 9:35

Throughout the gospel, Jesus healed the sick and set the captives free. The only criteria each person was required to have was faith. If by faith we are healed, can we also by faith be delivered from the temptation to overeat? I know that the Lord has all power, and it is at work in me and available to all those who believe.

The word also tells us that faith without works is dead. So if we believe, we have to act on what we believe. We have all heard the saying, "stepping out on faith."

To experience deliverance from anything, there is something required of us. We have to live a new way, think a new way, and eat in a new way.

I bought a Low Carb Cook Book last week. I know that I have to learn to cook healthy things that I enjoy in order to lose the weight and maintain my goal weight over time. When there are delicious foods that are good for me available,it decreases the need to make unhealthy choices. I am acting on faith.

I will learn a new way to cook:

_____

_____

_____

_____

_____

_____

_____

_____

_____

_____

_____

_____

_____

_____

_____

_____

_____

_____

_____

_____

_____

_____

_____

_____

_____

_____

Beloved, I wish above all things that you may prosper in all things and be in health, just as your soul prospers.
—3 John:2

Contrary to secular thinking, Christians are not deprived. In fact, our possibilities are actually limitless. Just as Satan tempted Jesus in the New Testament, he tempts us today. He wants us to think that we are missing out on something. But as we all know, he is a liar and very good at making things and situations seem better than they really are. If we look just beyond what he is offering, we will see it's really a trap. We can't continue to be fooled by the big empty box with the pretty red bow.

After losing weight in the past, I would look forward to eating all the foods I'd missed. When we are dieting, I know we will think about some of the foods we might enjoy when we are at our goal weight, but I used to plan many high calorie, fat-filled meals in my head. And once I felt comfortable with my size, I would start having my meals. Then I couldn't stop.

Dismissing my new eating habits is why it took me years to reach my goal. I was watching The Oprah Show a few weeks ago, and there was a man sharing his weight loss story. He'd lost 300 pounds in one year, which means in 11 years, I should have lost roughly 3,300 pounds!

Now when I reach my goal, I am looking forward to the image that I will see in the mirror and the results of my cholesterol test. My old approach—lose the weight and eat what you want—was not effective. That clearly does not work. My new approach is more like, learn how to eat healthy and carry that with you for the rest of your life.

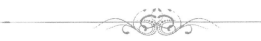

When I reach my goal, I look forward to:

The Lord will guide you continually, and satisfy your soul in drought, and strengthen your bones; you shall be like a watered garden, and be like a spring of water, whose waters do no fail.
—Isaiah 58:11 *(New King James Version)*

What would you be doing if you were at your goal weight? I ask this question because I think many of us hide behind our weight. Weight can cripple us in many ways. Just to name a few, it can keep us from realizing who we are in Christ, it can cause numerous health issues in our bodies, and it can be used as a excuse for us to avoid certain situations or opportunities.

Remember, our Heavenly Father is with us at all times and he keeps His promises.

If we are using weight as a shield or barrier, we can trade that option in for the Ultimate Protector. As we rest in Him, we can peel back the layers and soar on the wings of eagles.

When I get to my goal weight, I imagine things will change. I remember being a different person when I was smaller. I was less concerned about my appearance, less judgmental of other people, and I was more active. I am looking forward to shedding the extra pounds and rediscovering me.

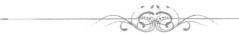

I use my weight as an excuse to avoid:

The wisdom of the prudent is to give thought to their ways, but the folly of the fool is deception.
—Proverbs 14:8 *(New International Version)*

I remember years ago there were bracelets and t-shirts that said: WWJD. We need to bring this back. A reminder to ask ourselves regularly, "what would Jesus do?" in this situation would save us a lot of headache. We should consider our steps.

What do I really want? I have to start asking myself that question. Yesterday, I wanted something sweet, but I was trying to be good and told myself, "no".

So as I was trying to avoid my sweet tooth, I ended up eating extra servings of spaghetti that night. I also ate bread, which I hadn't been doing. I believe if I had allowed myself to have a scoop of ice cream, the dinner would have gone a little differently. I would have had a normal portion of spaghettiand a scoop of ice cream. Instead, I added extra calories only to satisfy my craving for something sweet in the end.

As long as I am monitoring my portions, I am going to be honest with myself and deal with my cravings head on. Covering up a craving doesn't always work. If a salad won't work for me today, then I won't have one.

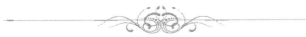

My extra calories are coming from:

_____

_____

_____

_____

_____

_____

_____

_____

_____

_____

_____

_____

_____

_____

_____

_____

_____

_____

_____

_____

_____

_____

_____

_____

The steps of the godly are directed by the Lord. He delights in every detail of their lives.
—Psalm 37:23 (NLT)

If we want a different result, it requires a different plan. We all know not to expect something new from the same old routine. If we want to live in the victory of the Lord, we must be willing to do a new thing. Only when we are willling to change and grow in Him can we experience all that God has for us.

It feels like I have reached another plateau in my weight loss. My plan is to increase the intensity of my workout. I'm trying a run/walk combination.

Instead of walking for 45 minutes, I will walk for three minutes and run for five minutes. I've been doing this now for a week, and it is not easy for me. I am not a runner.

In fact, I haven't run since junior high school. But when I go to the gym, it's hard not to stick with this new plan because it's working. I am noticing a difference. I am starting to lose again.

As I'm doing my run/walk though, there is usually a 120-pound person on the next treadmill running a fast sprint for 30+ minutes and barely breaking a sweat. I let that affect me for all of one minute, then I am in my own world of walking and running. I don't have time to feel embarrassed.

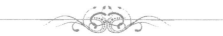

I can increase the intensity of my weight loss by:

_____

_____

_____

_____

_____

_____

_____

_____

_____

_____

_____

_____

_____

_____

_____

_____

_____

_____

_____

_____

_____

_____

_____

_____

_____

_____

_____

_____

God has not given us a spirit of fear, but of power and
of love and a sound mind.
—2 Timothy 1:7

We were created in the image of the almighty God, and I am living a defeated life?

Well, of course we will have challenges, but remembering whose spirit is alive in us, we have to know that we can handle anything that comes our way. We can live as if the King of Kings has our back, because He does.

We have house guests!!! This means: cakes, pies, macaroni and cheese, cornbread, potato salad, fried chicken, biscuits, bacon, and snacks galore. You name it, in the next three days it will be on the kitchen table. This is just the way our families are used to eating.

When we have guests, I usually eat what they eat. It's hard not to when you are helping to prepare the food and everyone eats together. I am getting stronger, but, if I am sitting next to you and you have some peach cobbler that I made, topped with ice cream, that's hard to resist. My goal this weekend is to watch my portions and get in plenty of water.

The more I think about it, with health issues related to diet and weight on the rise, maybe introducing a new way to eat and entertain when we have guests is long overdue. I know Patty LaBelle has a cook book that includes healthy southern recipes, I might have to pick that up.

I will address my food intake at a gathering or celebration by:

_____

_____

_____

_____

_____

_____

_____

_____

_____

_____

_____

_____

_____

_____

_____

_____

_____

_____

_____

_____

_____

_____

_____

_____

_____

_____

And let us not grow weary while doing good, for in due season we shall reap if we do not lose heart.
—Galatians 6:9 (*New King James Version*)

Wake up, wake up. We have a way of letting the good times rock us to sleep. When things are going well, we don't read the word as long, and we don't pray as hard.

The word tells us that we should pray without ceasing. Don't forget there is a war going on all around us.

The same truth applies to our weight loss journey. When we've dropped a few pounds, and we are starting to feel a little slimmer, we don't try as hard. We give in more to the desire to snack or skip a few workouts. Don't stop before you have received your full breakthrough.

I have reached many mini-goals. I have been so close to my goal I could taste it, only to slowly creep back up the scale. You know how disappointing that can be.

Well not this time. I am mad at the power I have given food in the past. I don't plan on doing that again.

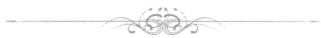

When I feel like stopping I will:

*A new commandment I give to you, that you love one another; as I have loved
you, that you also love one another.*
—John 13:34

When I was reading John 13:34, I wondered why the verse repeated the same phrase twice. Then I thought about it. That was for those of us who read it the first time and thought, "well, what if she…." The second time was to let us know that no criteria is required and nothing negates this command. Realistically, we don't have to like or approve of someone's actions, but we should be so filled with the love of Christ that no man can stomp it out.

Whether we admit it or not we need each other. God planned it that way. You encourage me, I encourage you. A kind word from a friend can make the difference.

Yesterday my husband said, "It looks like you're losing weight". He had a smile on his face, and that made my day. I plan to use that moment as fuel to motivate me throughout the week.

An encouraging word can make you feel so good. It also feels good to be an encourager. I am blessed when I am obediently a blessing to someone else.

I can be a blessing by:

_____

_____

_____

_____

_____

_____

_____

_____

_____

_____

_____

_____

_____

_____

_____

_____

_____

_____

_____

_____

_____

_____

_____

_____

_____

_____

_____

_____

_____

Be diligent to present yourself approved to God, a worker who does not need to be ashamed, rightly dividing the word of truth.
—2 Timothy 2:15 *(New King James Version)*

Let's be real, everyone knows their weakness. Take a good look at what that weakness is and develop a plan to deal with it. Very little creeps up on us without our knowing. If you are speeding down the highway, we know there is a chance the police would pull us over. We are disappointed, but not surprised.

The same thing applies to dieting. My weakness is snacking in the evenings and nibbling on food when I am cleaning the kitchen. If I could have avoided these two things, I would not be in this situation. To address these two weaknesses, I do three things. I buy healthy snacks that I like. I have my daughter help with the kitchen, and

I avoid the kitchen when ever possible. If it's after 7:00 p.m., I have no real reason to go into that room. If I spend extra time in there, who am I kidding? I know what's going to happen.

When I came face to face with my weakness, I put myself in control. As long as I was ignoring what was really going on, I could not experience victory over it.

My true weakness is:

Praise be to the God and Father of our Lord Jesus Christ, the Father
of compassion and the God of all comfort, who comforts us in all our troubles,
so that we can comfort those in any trouble with the comfort we ourselves
have received from God.
—2 Corinthians 1:3,4 *(New International Version)*

I lost someone who was very important to me. What a way to be re-minded just how fragile and privileged life is. Not just your life, but the life of those around you. We really don't have time to give priority to frivolous things.

Life is meant to be enjoyed and lived with a purpose. Are we wasting it? Right now, weight loss seems so petty. The gift of life is so precious, and what do we do with it?

We use it to make nonlife choices, choices that are destructive and not edifying to our Lord, to ourselves, and to our life.

Obesity is crippling the lives of so many people. Now more than ever I feel the need to put this weight loss goal behind me and share my story with the hope of helping someone else experience the victory God has for us. Life is precious and living it is so much more important than... food.

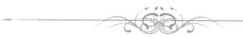

Remembering how precious life is, I will:

_____

_____

_____

_____

_____

_____

_____

_____

_____

_____

_____

_____

_____

_____

_____

_____

_____

_____

_____

_____

_____

_____

_____

_____

_____

_____

_____

_____

Teach me, O Lord, to follow your decrees; then I will keep them
to the end. Give me understanding, and I will keep your law
and obey it with all my heart. Direct me in the path of your commands,
for there I find delight.
—Psalm 119:33-35 *(New International Version)*

We have all stepped ahead of God and gone the wrong way, only because our prayer wasn't answered in our time. God knows what's best for us. When you think about it, do you really want to be outside of His appointed time? Patience is a virtue.

Practice makes perfect. It may be a grade school cliché, but it is a very practical concept. We know the saying—if you practice something long enough, you can become really good at it. The challenge isn't just doing something, but doing it long enough. "I tried working out last week and I don't like it". That definitely is not long enough.

I remember when I first started working out. It felt uncomfortable. I was one of the biggest people there. I got tired quick, and I was more concerned with the other one million and one things I could be doing. I had to push myself to workout.

Now I work out religiously, and I actually look forward to it. To look at my technique I am sure you wouldn't say, "that looks perfect". But, I do have perfect attendance.

It would be easy to just sit around and never do anything that requires much effort but what would I accomplish? Practice, no matter how we look. Practice, even if we don't feel like it. Practice makes perfect.

I will practice:

_____

_____

_____

_____

_____

_____

_____

_____

_____

_____

_____

_____

_____

_____

_____

_____

_____

_____

_____

_____

_____

_____

_____

_____

_____

_____

I will sprinkle clean water on you, and you will be clean;
I will cleanse you from all your impurities and from
all your idols.
—Ezekiel 36:25 *(New King James Version)*

Wow, water is an amazing thing. The scriptures refer to water in many terms, to name a few: cleansing, renewing and rebirth. Water is a spiritual symbol of life. Moses was put in the water to preserve his life. The "Red Sea" is a testimony that God will fight your battles. Baptism confirms that we can begin again.

Over the last several weeks, water has become the key component in my journey to weight loss. I have been getting in eight glasses, and it is making more of a difference than I expected. I am used to drinking for taste, not health, so this is a big change for me.

Water has helped to curb my appetite. I have lost more weight, and it has increased my energy level. When you think about it, it makes sense. The more water I get in, the less room in my stomach for other things. The more water I get in, the more my body is cleansed of impurities.

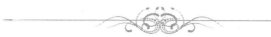

My plan for increasing my water intake is:

_____

_____

_____

_____

_____

_____

_____

_____

_____

_____

_____

_____

_____

_____

_____

_____

_____

_____

_____

_____

_____

_____

_____

_____

For wisdom will enter your heart,
and knowledge will be pleasant to your soul.
—Proverbs 2:10 *(New International Version)*

For me, keeping a journal is one of those peculiar things. I am a very private person.

In fact, when my husband bought me this journal, I remember how much I appreciated the thought, but I had no plans of using it. Now look, I am not only using it, but I am sharing it with who ever would be interested in reading it.

Writing in this journal has truly been a blessing beyond words. I have never been so focused on my health goals. Journaling has given me clarity and a voice to express my thoughts. It has given me the opportunity to not only develop a plan, but it has also been a tool of encouragement and accountability.

I will keep journaling even after I reach my weight loss goal. I don't think you ever get too old to grow and learn new things. I wonder what the title of my next journal will be, "A Christian Woman's Journal to..."

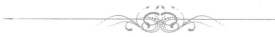

Journaling has allowed me to:

_____

_____

_____

_____

_____

_____

_____

_____

_____

_____

_____

_____

_____

_____

_____

_____

_____

_____

_____

_____

_____

_____

_____

_____

_____

_____

WEEK FORTY-NINE

Praise the Lord, O my soul; all my inmost being,
praise His holy name. Praise the Lord, O my soul,
and forget not all His benefits-
—Psalm 103:1 *(New International Version)*

What a great feeling!! Most of the things in my closet fit. My weight loss has made me feel better about myself. I went to a party yesterday, and I actually enjoyed getting dressed. When normally I dread the chore of finding something that will fit, I had many choices to choose from.

Did you know that your feet can get smaller, too? I had many shoes that I didn't wear because they were too uncomfortable. Well, last night I wore a pair of boots that I had never worn before. I could always get them on, but the thought of wearing them for an extended period of time seemed painful. Not only was I able to wear them, but they felt fine all evening.

Sometimes we can get comfortable in being uncomfortable, and we end up giving up on doing anything about it. I thank God for the mind to trust Him and believe that I can do all things...

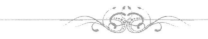

I am not giving up because:

_____

_____

_____

_____

_____

_____

_____

_____

_____

_____

_____

_____

_____

_____

_____

_____

_____

_____

_____

_____

_____

_____

_____

_____

_____

_____

_____

_____

_____

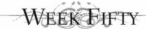

But when he asks, he must believe and not doubt,
because he who doubts is like a wave of the sea, blown and tossed
by the wind.
—James 1:6 *(New International Version)*

When I started working out, I was walking on the treadmill. I remember that being hard for me. Then I started a run/walk combination, and that was again a stretch for me. Now, I am running for 25 minutes! The other day I was at the gym and feeling confident. I just decided to try running for a longer period of time, and I lasted for 25 minutes. In the past, I was so convinced that I was not a runner, that I would never have even attempted to do this.

So much of what we do is tied to what we think. I never thought I could run, so I didn't. I never thought I could get down to a size 8, so I never tried. I never thought I could be a water drinker, so I always bought soda.

If we don't believe it can happen, how hard will we work to make it happen? Having faith is the start of any good thing that we might achieve in life. Doubt and unbelief have no place in the mind of a Christian. I will believe in myself and the ability that I have through Christ.

I believe:

_____

_____

_____

_____

_____

_____

_____

_____

_____

_____

_____

_____

_____

_____

_____

_____

_____

_____

_____

_____

_____

_____

_____

_____

_____

_____

_____

_____

_____

WEEK FIFTY-ONE

The blessing of the Lord makes one rich, and He adds
no sorrow to it.
—Proverbs 10:22 *(New King James Version)*

What a blessing to be so close to a goal that has been a long time coming.

In the beginning, it seemed impossible because I had failed so many times before. I had to rethink this thing and figure out why I'd failed in the pastand honestly address those issues. I had lost focus on what's important. We can get so caught up in meeting deadlines and staying on task that we neglect ourselves and those things that matter the most. The world offers so much, and it is our responsibility to consider what is available and make godly and healthy lifestyle choices.

Trusting in the Lord—it's not just a religious statement or motto. Trust is a verb, so it depicts action. Because we trust in Him, we live by His word, not by the ways of the world. Overindulging in nothing, sensibly nourishing our soul, our mind and our body. His instructions for this life are very clear, when they're not clouded by outside influences.

During your struggling, think about how an antibiotic works. We may not see the effects of it right away, but if we keep taking it we will see results. When it seems like your weight loss has comes to a slow crawl and your level of effort is there, the results of your effort will eventually manifest. Stay encouraged.

When I look back at my journey, I have no regrets. It was hard work, but I am glad I did it. There were days when I wanted to quit, but thank God for endurance.

I am who He says I am. I will never forget that or let anyone or anything, defy WHOSE I am.

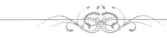

God says I am:

_____

_____

_____

_____

_____

_____

_____

_____

_____

_____

_____

_____

_____

_____

_____

_____

_____

_____

_____

_____

_____

_____

_____

_____

_____

_____

_____

_____

_____

_____

Peace I leave with you. My peace I give to you, not as the world gives do I give to you. Let not your heart be troubled, neither let it be afraid.
—John 14:27 *(New International Version)*

As women we are wonderful creations of God, not to be defined by images seen in magazines or on television, but defined by the image in which we were made. Of course, we all have looked in the mirror and not been ecstatic by what we saw, but does that give us a reason to be critical of ourselves to the point of self-destruction? Just as God loved us while we were yet in sin, we can love ourselves even as we are evolving--being at peace with who we are and who we can become. Yes, God gave us His peace and at some point we gave it back, replacing it with stress, anxiety, and depression. We decided to trust in our own understanding, to walk in our strength, or to forget to put on the whole armor of God.

A calm place of complete submissiveness. This is how I define peace. Arriving at such a place does not suggest that I will not experience struggle, disappointment, or moments of personal weakness. But what a joy to rely and rest in HIM. There is victory for every aspect of our life in the word of the Lord.

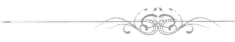

I am victorious because:

_____

_____

_____

_____

_____

_____

_____

_____

_____

_____

_____

_____

_____

_____

_____

_____

_____

_____

_____

_____

_____

_____

_____

_____

_____

_____

_____

_____

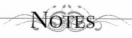

NOTES

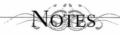

NOTES

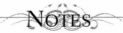

NOTES

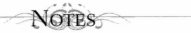

NOTES

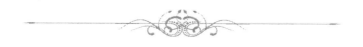

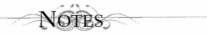

NOTES

Also available from The Elevator Group Faith:
A Christian Woman's Journal to Weight Loss Affirmation Cards,
by Patricia Thomas: 53 cards to reinforce the scripture and reflections in
A Christian Woman's Journal to Weight Loss. Price: $15.95

Coming in summer 2009 from the Elevator Group Faith:
*Creativity for Christians: How to Write your Story and Stories
of Overcoming from the Members of One Special Church*,
by Sheilah Vance with Rev. Felicia Howard:
We are made overcomers by the blood of the lamb and the word of our testimony (Rev. 12:11). Everyone has a story to tell. Learn how to tell yours.
50% writing workshop. 50% stories of victory. 100% inspiring.

Also available from The Elevator Group:
Land Mines, a novel, by Sheilah Vance.

Journaling Through the Land Mines, by Sheilah Vance:
a companion journal to Land Mines.

Chasing the 400, a novel, by Sheilah Vance.

For more information about any of the items above,
visit www.TheElevatorGroup.com.

To order any of the items above, contact
Atlas Books Distribution,
30 Amberwood Parkway, Ashland, Ohio 44805
or place your order toll-free at 1-800-247-6553
or on-line at www.atlasbooks.com.

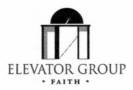

ELEVATOR GROUP
• FAITH •

Helping People Rise Above™